Tales of the Exam Room Volume 2: **Medical Horror Stories**

Copyright © 2021 Scott Kemp

ISBN: 978-1-7361598-6-6 (Paperback)

ISBN: 978-1-7361598-7-3 (EBook)

Second Edition 2021.

Credits:

Book Cover and Formatting by farhanshahid101

Obsidian Wolf Publishing

PO Box 1086 Salem, UT 84653

Contents

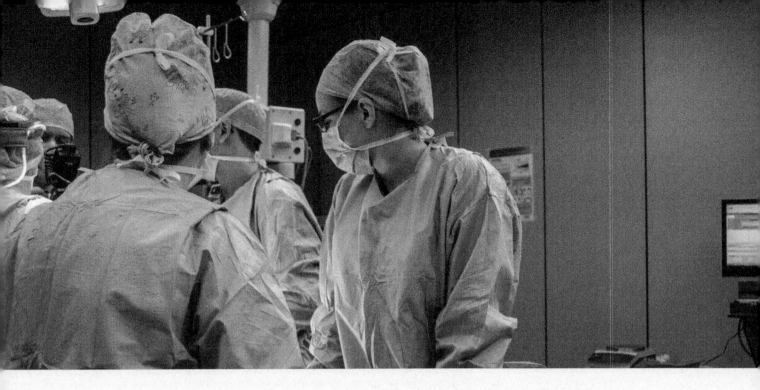

Introduction

Medical Horror Stories: Tales of the Exam Room – Vol 2.

These stories are personal and often true in nature but have been changed slightly to protect the privacy or the experience of a story. In medicine, we often love our patients beyond the common understanding, and we love medicine. We strive to help patients whenever possible, though that is not always an option. Sometimes the patient is their own worst enemy.

In this book, we try to help the readers understand the love for both the patient and medicine. The art of medicine is seldom black and white. There are many reasons why it is called "practicing" medicine. Sometimes, decisions are made in a split moment, and what works for one patient, may or may not work for another.

Patients are people. They are not always defined by their medical conditions. But some stories touch us in ways that unless you were there, it is hard to understand. Furthermore, not everyone thinks the same. Some people will leave the hospital AMA (Against Medical Advice) and refuse procedures that could save their lives.

Other patients will self-sabotage or misunderstand what is being recommended. These stories try to capture the lives and choices of several different individuals.

As mentioned in Volume One - This is a fictional piece and is mainly for entertainment. Our goal is to allow you to see into the world of medicine and some of the bizarre encounters that have happened. If your story happens to line up exactly with ours, trust me – we are not that good, and it's probably more of a coincidence. There are some medical truths and teachings that have been added for the readers' benefit.

Feel free to Join Us for additional medical stories at examroomtales.com

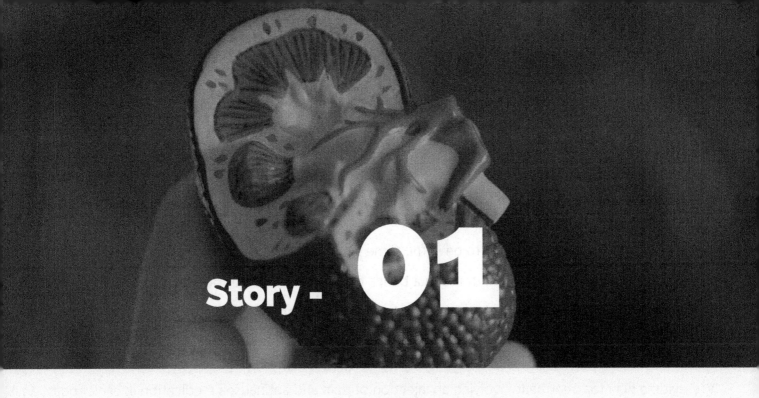

Reoccurring Kidney Stones

I was seeing a patient, Jeffrey, that I knew pretty well for reoccurring kidney stones and worsening pain over the past few days. Coincidently, this was the third time in the previous three weeks that I saw Jeffrey for the same complaint. He had been my patient for the last seven or eight years, maybe longer. I had seen him the day he was sent for surgery on his appendix about three years ago. I had also seen him for a few colds and ear infections over the years.

Jeffrey had a well-documented history of kidney stones, including previous treatment with medications and lithotripsy. Lithotripsy is a medical procedure that uses shock waves or a laser to break small stones in the kidneys so that they can pass.

The first two times I saw him, he was sweating, grimacing in pain, and had blood in his urine. I had recommended that he get a CT to evaluate the stones, their sizes, and their numbers. I tried at length to convince him to get additional testing. Jeffrey just told me that he didn't have the insurance for such an evaluation because he was no longer on his parent's insurance plan. In each of the previous visits, I prescribed something for pain and another medication to help the stones a better chance to pass.

In the exam room, Jeffrey appeared to be in the same situation as before. I was frustrated that he didn't have a way to get better treatment. I ran through a bunch of questions and performed an examination. This time, the pain was on the opposite side, his left flank, which isn't uncommon. He looked miserable -cold, pale, clammy. I feared that he was going to throw up in my exam room.

We made a plan for treatment involving an injection of pain and antinausea medication in clinic today, an IV for fluids, and some medicine to go home with. We moved Jeffrey to a different exam room, better situated for IV fluids and laying down. I told him that he still needed to provide a urine sample. I also wanted him to use a special strainer to collect the stone. He said that he would, and I left to find my nurse and gather the necessary supplies.

Kidney stones are quite common and can be excruciatingly painful. If you get one stone, you are at risk of getting another and another. There are some environmental factors that can cause stones, such as food, soda, dehydration, and more. There is likely a genetic factor as well. Some unlucky patients get stones after stones, no matter what we do. I was starting to feel that Jeffrey might be in this category.

When a stone is created in the kidney - it usually passes to the bladder and out the body. That process can be painful. But sometimes, the stone(s) is too large and can't escape the kidney. When this happens, the pain can be intense. That is why a CT exam and lithotripsy are necessary.

With my nurse's help, it wasn't hard to grab the supplies that we needed, including the shot for pain, and head back to the exam room. As my nurse and I stepped back into the room, we were shocked at what we found. Jeffrey hadn't heard us, and he was talking on the phone. It felt weird standing there and listening. He stood near the sink, and he had something in his hand. His pants were down near the floor.

He said, "I'll have the pills in an hour. Don't worry about it."

Jeffrey was doing something that we couldn't really see, and normally, I would be worried that he was sick or something. But the way Jeffrey was acting and how he was talking, he was anything but sick. He was almost laughing when he said, "I got this whole thing covered."

My nurse and I stepped closer.

Jeffrey placed something on top of the sink, but he still didn't know that we were in the room. I recognized it immediately as a paper clip partially bent so that one side was open. There was blood on the paper clip.

"What in the world is happening here?" My nurse asked.

Jeffrey jumped as if he had been caught by surprise. He turned around, and his face started turning bright red.

To my horror, I realized what he was doing. To get blood in his urine, he was sticking the paper clip, purposely, into the tip of his penis. He was doing this because blood is one of the more essential symptoms of kidney stones.

In my practice, I really try to be nonjudgmental towards any of my patients and give them the benefit of the doubt. Over the years, I have learned that not every patient tells the truth, but additionally, most patients aren't trying to deceive. But what Jeffrey was doing was blatantly clear.

"I can totally explain," Jeffrey said.

I was shocked and saddened at the extreme measures he was willing to take. I had been tricked, and he was caught right in the act.

"I think we all know what is going on here. You probably should leave," I said.

He quickly apologized, dressed as he grabbed all his items, and ran from our clinic. I haven't seen Jeffrey since.

I would have never imagined the lengths someone would go through to get pain medications. These days, I am a little more cautious, but I can't let one person's mistakes affect how I treat all the rest of my patients. You can't assume that every patient you see is drug-seeking.

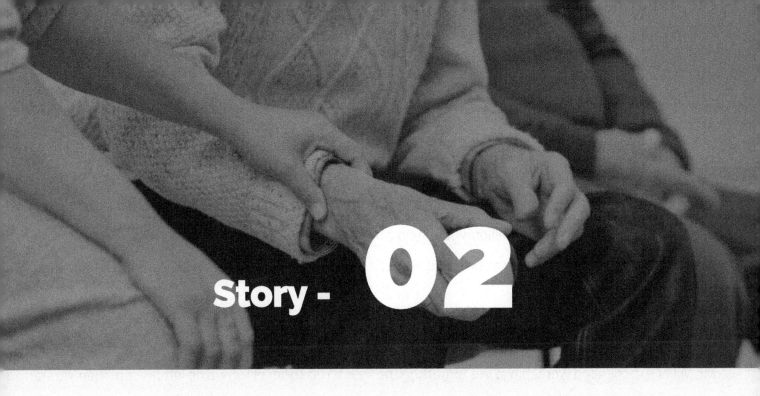

Story - 02

A Swing and a Miss - Nursing Home Style

Dementia, especially in the elderly, is a combination of unexpected changes with unintended consequences. This is often for the families as much as for the patient themselves. Working with these patients, you never really know how each encounter or episode will go. You need to be ready for the unexpected.

Dementia is a heartbreaking thing to watch, especially if you have known the person for many years. They become people that they weren't previously. As a medical professional, I often want to explain to family members with what they should expect. But you can never adequately prepare loved ones for what they are about to witness as the disease progresses.

My story is about an older gentleman that I have known for several years. Mr. Miller was in his late seventies when he started experiencing dementia symptoms. Up until that point, he was living in a care center -on his own and doing quite well.

Mr. Miller hadn't driven in a few years, and before his symptoms became worse, his daughter picked him up twice a week to go to the grocery store and out to lunch. Other friends would stop by and visit him. He could cook and clean on his own. Mr. Miller would help other residents and was very kind. He would attend church services and bible study as often as he could. His wife had passed away when Mr. Miller was in his sixties.

When his dementia symptoms kicked in, things went downhill. It wasn't long before his children were forced to put him in a more skilled nursing home, one with locked doors and twenty-four-hour care. The first changes Mr. Miller experienced were things like forgetting the keys to his room or where he left his cup. Then, he started forgetting where his room was or where he was living. Then the faces of his family were no longer those that he remembered.

The interesting thing was that he could remember the year 1970 without any problems. He would continuously sing three songs: My Sweet Lord by George Harrison, The Long and Winding Road by the Beatles, and Bridge over Troubled Water by Simon and Garfunkel. You could ask him to sing these three songs, and he remembered them perfectly. He also loved and quoted the television show MASH without any problems.

As I previously mentioned, his wife, Mrs. Miller, had passed previously. She had died of breast cancer. Mr. Miller had pictures of her and stories and stories to tell about her. Soon Mr. Miller's stories changed, as did the names that he used. They were all about his wife, but he couldn't remember her name and often slipped in a different name. It was sad to watch.

About six months into the new nursing home, Mr. Miller had a week I'll never forget.

It first started on a weekend night. I think the facility was serving chicken or something. Mr. Miller wanted anything to eat but chicken. He was adamant and wouldn't listen to what anyone else said. We were feeding about thirty other residents, and the food had been prepared in advance. Mr. Miller was directed to the fridge, where there were a few different options, leftovers from lunch and the night before. He refused to move and demanded that all the food be brought to his spot. The plate of chicken was pushed away, along with lunch from earlier in the day. The nursing assistant passing out the food, pointed to the fridge, and moved onto the next patient who needed their dinner. She said, "Go find something else if you want."

A few minutes later, Mr. Miller screamed, "Order me a pizza."

This set off a few of the other residents because they also wanted pizza. We tried explaining that chicken was what was for dinner, and they would try to put pizza on the menu for later in the week.

Mr. Miller went ballistic and reached over and picked up his plate of chicken, throwing it across the room. As if in slow motion, it sailed through the air and landed in the middle of a group of women. Mr. Miller then reached for the two plates next to him and threw them as well. This unleashed the biggest food fight I've ever seen. Every resident got hit with food and threw whatever they could find.

I'll never forget seeing old ladies in wheelchairs throwing food.

A few days later, Mr. Miller became convinced that his wheelchair had been stolen. He didn't ask any staff members to help. Instead, he went around to all the other residents, about fifteen, who had wheelchairs and knocked them out of their wheelchairs to get a better look. Luckily, no one was seriously injured.

When the staff members finally caught up with Mr. Miller, they tried to listen to Mr. Millers' explanation. He was ranting and raving about his missing wheelchair that his wife had gotten him for Christmas a few months ago. It took several long minutes for the staff member to explain that Mr. Miller had never used a wheelchair once in his life. Therefore, how did someone steal his wheelchair when he didn't own one.

The third episode was from a male technician that was helping Mr. Miller shower. This happens several times a week. Each resident has an individual room, but some do share a bathroom with another resident. In this case, Mr. Miller has his own room and bathroom. He has an open shower with a rail and handles, which helps prevent falls.

Mr. Miller often gets distracted or refuses to shower and needs someone to help him. On this day, the male technician was helping Mr. Miller, but Mr. Miller was in a foul mood. He wanted no part of getting out of bed, dressing, and especially didn't want to shower.

But Mr. Miller had soiled himself and required a shower and new clothing. Halfway through, the technician noticed that something changed in Mr. Miller's behavior. It was like a fog over his memory had vanished. Mr. Miller's mind became clear, and he knew exactly where he was, and he didn't like it one bit. This didn't seem to improve his mood, and he started fighting with the technician. The problem was that Mr. Miller still had conditioner in his hair that needed to be washed out before he was done. The technician tried frantically to rinse Mr. Miller's hair. This made things worse, and that was when Mr. Miller attacked. He balled up his fist and shot out at the groin of the technician.

Luckily the technician was fast enough and jumped out of the way. Mr. Miller, however, slipped on the water and lost his footing. He stumbled forward and fell. The technician jumped and luckily caught Mr. Miller before he hit the ground. But soon, everyone in the shower was soaking wet.

Mr. Miller said, "Your fault here, you pervert."

The technician helped Mr. Miller out of the shower, dried him off, and started getting him dressed. By this time, Mr. Miller had forgotten everything that had just happened. His focus was on getting back into bed and watching some television. During the dressing process, Mr. Miller was suddenly kind and helpful. He was chatting as if he and the technicians were best friends.

Needless to say, Mr. Miller had a really tough week. Dementia can do that to you. I share these episodes to help you have a better understanding of some of the difficult times that many elderly, residents, and nursing staff go through to care for those with similar conditions. Nursing homes, in general, can be very emotional and challenging.

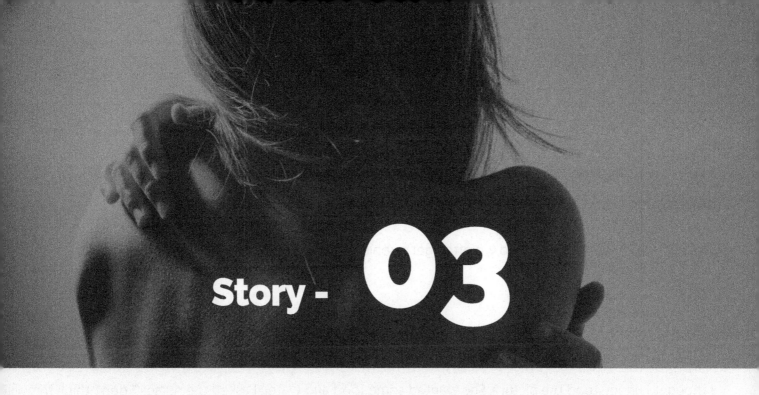

Story - 03

The Rash on my Back that Won't Go Away

I was volunteering, and do so regularly, for a homeless clinic in the inner cities. We have a bus that drives around to a few different locations. People, not always homeless, stand in line until it was their turn. My fifth or sixth patient of the day was an older lady, probably in her late fifties. It was at least seventy-five degrees out; however, she was wearing a sweater and a jacket.

As is customary, she filled out her pre-screening packet. She was on medication for blood pressure, cholesterol, schizophrenia, depression, and anxiety. She needed a refill of each of these. It was easy to get them reordered. She also wanted to have blood work for HIV, Hepatitis, Diabetes, and other general blood tests.

At the window of the bus, I reviewed her paperwork and her requests. Her examination would be pretty basic. At the end of the initial screening, she added, "I've also got this rash on my back that won't go away."

I had the nurse call her back to one of the exam rooms on the bus as I wrote out the refills for her medications.

When I was finished, I stepped towards the room. The nurse caught my attention. She said, "The lady is sweating like crazy. She won't take off her jacket or sweater."

The bus was air-conditioned, and we often get people who just want a break from the heat.

"That's fine. Is she in the room?"

"No," the nurse said. "She needed to use the bathroom. I'm also getting her some snacks and some water."

I thought I understood the picture. She wanted some food and water. I asked the nurse, "I don't think this will take long, but will you be my chaperone?" Our nurses help facilitate things, as well as to provide a level of protection for the patient as well as for myself. You can never be too careful.

"No problem."

When I entered, the smell was overwhelming. I shared a glance with the nurse but wasn't overly concerned.

"Hello Mrs. Simmons. How are you feeling?"

"Pretty good."

"I have your medication refills. I'm going to look at your rash, and at the end, we will get started on that blood work."

"Sounds good," Mrs. Simmons replied.

I asked, "How long have you had this rash on your back?"

"Three or four weeks."

"Does it itch? Can you see it?"

"It doesn't itch. But it is so very painful. Sometimes it feels like it burns, and other times it feels like I am being stabbed in my back. I don't own a mirror, so I haven't been able to see it."

"Are you homeless?"

"Yes. I was in a shelter until about a month ago. Recently, I got approved for some governmental housing. I'll be able to move into an apartment at the end of the week."

"That's great to hear. Are you allergic to any medications?"

"Not that I know of."

"Is it alright if we look at your back?"

"Do you have to?"

"It would help us a lot.

"I guess. But I'll need help taking off my clothes."

"My nurse can help with that."

The outer jacket was pretty easy to remove. My nurse pointed to the back of the sweatshirt underneath, which had a large stain on the back. It appeared as if she'd been wearing it for several days. There were more stains on the front that looked like food. My eyes were drawn to a stain on her back. It was as large as a basketball and was still slightly wet as if it had rained recently. It was hot out, so I was hoping the stain was from sweat.

My nurse and I helped Mrs. Simmons out of her sweater and was surprised to find that she had on several shirts underneath. The instant the sweater was removed, the smell in the bus worsened and ripened. Each of her T-shirts seemed to be plastered and stuck to her back.

I asked, "Has the rash been draining any fluids?"

"I think so."

"When did that start?"

"About a week after the rash first appeared. I found that the back of my shirt was wet. It was worse after sitting or lying down. I didn't have a way to clean my back, so I just added another shirt. I figured it would stop being wet sooner or later. After that one got wet, I added my sweater and then my jacket. I just didn't know what else to do."

It took us about twenty minutes to remove the remaining t-shirts. We had to soak areas with hydrogen peroxide, cut pieces of the shirt. When the last layers of the T-shirt were removed, I was shocked by what I saw.

"Did you have blisters on your back?"

"Maybe." Mrs. Simmons shrugged. "I couldn't really see them. I could feel them squish back and forth whenever I rubbed up against something. My skin burned so bad."

"I think I know exactly what happened."

"You do?" she asked, perplexed. "Can you fix it?"

"We will get you all the help you need," I said.

My nurse whispered, "How could a rash get so bad?"

"I've never seen something get this bad."

Mrs. Simmons's entire skin was inflamed and red. There were areas with clear drainage, but there were also areas of skin breakdown and purulent discharge. It took several minutes to clean the skin.

"Did I get this rash because I was dirty?" Mrs. Simmons asked.

"Not really. Actually, what you had is called Shingles. But not being able to clean it might have made it worse."

"I've never heard of it."

"It comes from a virus, actually, the same one that causes chickenpox. But, when you get older, you get these huge blisters in one area of the body instead of all over. Does that make sense?"

"I think so."

"The problem, in your case, is that because of the size of the area and that you are homeless, I think that on top of the shingles, a bacterial infection also got into your skin. In fact, it's pretty serious. You have pus over your entire back. There are large pockets of sores and such. We need to send you to the hospital for IV antibiotics and treatment."

"I can't afford that."

"Ma'am. The hospital will work that out with you. The problem is that your infection is so bad that if you don't get treatment, you could die."

"Are you sure it's that bad?" she asked.

"Completely sure."

Neither my nurse nor I had never seen such a serious case of secondary bacterial infection. We gave her a gown that we had and several extra shirts for after she left the hospital. We called an ambulance to make sure she went to the hospital, and didn't refuse. It was a wonder that Mrs. Simmons was walking, talking, or eating anything at all. She was extremely sick.

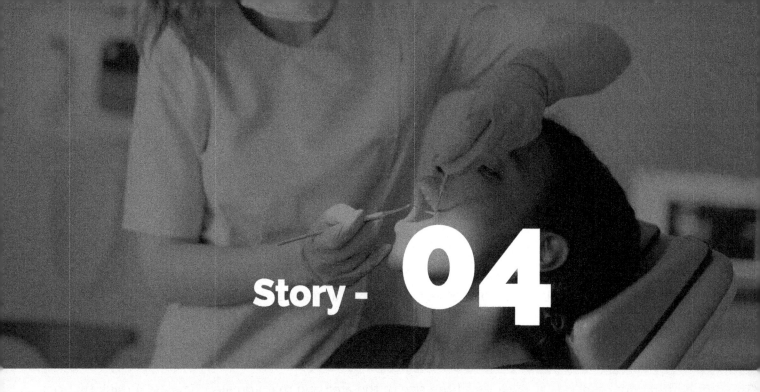

Story - 04

Dental Pain and Infection with a Surprising Cause

First and foremost, it is crucial to understand that I am not a dentist. However, I visit many places inside this country as well as outside, where traditional dental services are not always available. This means that I treat dental problems and emergencies when called upon. In one such case, the patient was having dental pain along with an infection. Over time, I learned that the causes of both were quite surprising and horrific.

I was on a medical mission visiting several small villages in a different country, and I had been in the country for almost three weeks. This village was one of the final destinations on our trip. I ended up staying in this area for about six days and was treating a wide variety of medical, mental health, and dental problems. I had a handful of nurses with me and several other medical personal. We worked hard to provide a small measure of hope inside this village.

The temperature in this region was hot and humid, and it had been a semi-difficult journey to get to this point. In some of these trips, it seems like the clinics and transportation can go smoothly, or everything can go wrong. So far, we had undoubtedly traveled the more difficult path.

It took several hours to set up the clinic and get things ready for the next day. We would set up a triage program lead by my nurses. I would end up seeing only patients that required medicine or had more serious concerns. Mr. D was my third patient of the morning. Through a translator, he explained to me that he had been having tooth pains for years. Two years ago, he had three of his teeth pulled. That had helped the pain until it returned six months ago.

I performed a full head-to-toe exam, leaving the teeth for last. I could see that Mr. D had rather good dentition, all considering. He was missing the previously mentioned teeth. Mr. D pointed to the opposite side of the mouth, showing me what was causing him pain. He described, in very energetic details, what he was dealing with. The village does not have fluoride in their water to help with teeth, and they don't have toothpaste to use every day. This patient would be lucky to see a dentist five times in his life.

The tooth that Mr. D pointed to was partially broken. There was a small area of blackness on the lower edge of the tooth near the gum line. This is also not uncommon. He had minimal swelling, no redness, and some pain when drinking water. With a broken tooth, I was worried about an exposed nerve root. On exam, there was a minimal amount of pain.

I felt I had three options: First, give some NSAID like ibuprofen alone and see how he did. Second, along with ibuprofen, I could add an antibiotic. Third, I could just pull the tooth. I decided to try just ibuprofen. Mr. D liked the idea of trying to save the tooth. He was more than willing to be conservative about his treatment, knowing that I would still be around for the next few days. If I were leaving the same day, I would've just pulled the tooth. I told him that he could stop by anytime in the next few days if he had more problems.

Two days later, he returned by the clinic for another evaluation. This time, his face had started to swell, especially on the same side as the dental pain. His pain had now skyrocketed, and he had trouble sitting still. In the last six hours, he had been forced to stopped eating because of the symptoms. This time, on the exam, there was redness and swelling near the tooth in question. The gums appeared very tender. We gave him twenty pills of an antibiotic to take over the next several days. The village did not have a local pharmacy for their medications, and they relied on our help.

Day six arrived, and I was mostly packed to leave and head back home. We had seen over half the village and had taken care of many problems. Everyone was so kind and humble and thanked us repeatedly. As I was finishing up, Mr. D stopped back by. I was hoping that I would see him again and hear that things were getting better. That was not the case.

The swelling was about the same from my standpoint. Mr. D was frustrated because he had thought that things were getting better. In fact, he had eaten dinner the previous night without any pain. When he woke up this morning, the pain and swelling were back.

The only option remaining was to pull the tooth. I explained this to Mr. D. More than anything, he wanted this entire problem resolved. I grabbed some equipment and a nurse to help. I tried numbing the gums just near the tooth. Using clean forceps, the tooth was removed with little difficulty. The patient's gums started to bleed a little, but nothing significant.

I placed the tooth in a small white container. After getting some gauze to help the bleeding, the patient asked to look at the tooth. I was guessing that he wanted to keep it, so I started cleaning the tooth when something began moving from within the tooth, on the bottom side.

I was taken by surprise and I admit that I jumped back a step or two. A few seconds later, I reexamined the tooth, and I instantly recognized what was happening. The inner portion of the tooth had decayed, which created a hollow portion of the tooth. Inside this hollow portion were five or six white worms. They were wriggling back and forth. They were so tiny.

I next performed an exam on Mr. D, and sure enough, there was a small hole in the gums where the tooth had been removed. I cleaned out the area and dislodged two additional worms. The patient's entire mouth was cleaned with a strong mouth wash for the next several days. Mr. D was ordered to continue taking the antibiotic and the additional medications.

In the end, he was bound to get better. I was extremely happy that Mr. D came back one last time. I would hate to know what would've happened if the tooth hadn't been removed.

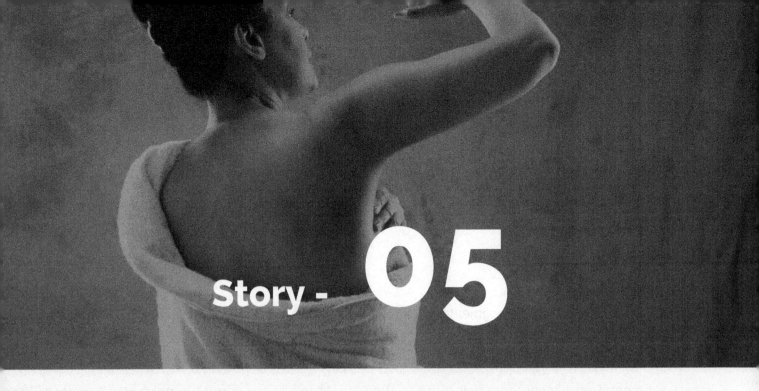

Breast Implants Gone Wrong

Before walking into the exam room, I was warned that the patient inside, likely homeless, was sick and hadn't showered in several days. My nurse explained that she would only speak with the provider about why she was in the Emergency Room. My guess was that she was embarrassed. Many people come to the emergency room with embarrassing stories, situations, and medical concerns.

The patient sat on the bed with a dazed look on her face. She was slouching down, like she had her head in her hands, appearing so small. She was pale, sweating, and clearly uncomfortable.

From the doorway, I said, "Hello. Thanks for coming to the Emergency Room. My name is Doctor Favors. How can I help you?"

She replied by saying, "Oh, thank you very much, doctor, for seeing me. I'm Pam, and I'm sorry that it has come to this. I'm in really bad shape. It is kind of embarrassing, but I need your help."

"Are you injured, or are you sick?"

"Kind of both."

"When did this happen?"

"Things all started with a breast augmentation a few months ago. It has quickly gone from bad to worse."

I have to admit that I wasn't expecting this sort of explanation. You don't see many homeless people with breast augmentation. I knew there was more to the story than just her current appearance. Admittedly, she appeared that she had been on the streets for years. Her clothes were ragged, torn, and she hadn't had a good night's sleep in months. She had some boils on her arms and some track marks. She was gaunt and sickly.

I said, "I am sure we can help you. Are you homeless?"

"I am," Pam admitted. "But it wasn't always this way."

"What medical problems are you currently having?"

"I normally don't take any medications. I don't have any chronic problems like high blood pressure or diabetes. But I'm pretty sure I have an infection."

"Treating an infection is something that we see a lot of. What makes you think you have an infection, and how did this start with breast surgery?"

She started her story by saying, "I had breast surgery about six months ago. My boyfriend at the time wanted it done. He was willing to pay for it. Surgery was a breeze, and I was really happy to have it done as well as the outcome. It looked amazing. I had minimal pain and swelling. I only missed a day or two of work. At the time, I was driving a two-year-old red corvette. It was so beautiful. I was living in my own apartment and had a steady job. I know that how I look now is a far cry from just a few months ago."

"So, what happened?"

"Here's where it gets interesting," Pam explained. "About three weeks after surgery, I was driving to work, and I was in a car accident, that wasn't even my fault. I was stopped at a red light and was rear-ended by a work truck. I'm not even sure he braked before hitting me."

"That doesn't sound good."

"Hit from behind, and I smacked the person in front of me. I got whiplash and somehow hit my steering wheel extremely hard. An ambulance was called, and I was sent to the hospital. I was so worried about my ribs and my neck. I think I even had a cut on my forehead. I spent two or three nights in the hospital. They ran several tests. Luckily, I just had a concussion and whiplash, but no broken bones. They checked out my implants and told me that everything seemed to be alright. They suggested I return to my surgeon for a check-up. They gave me some pain medication and released me from the hospital."

"That sounds like a terrible experience."

"It was horrible and very painful. That accident sent my life into a tailspin."

"What do you mean?"

"I have known for years, even been in and out of rehab. But I have an addiction problem. I was doing so well for the last few years. It didn't take long, but after only a few days on the pain medications, I lost control. I returned to my doctor and told him that the pain was severe. He quickly refilled my pain medications. When that didn't work, I found some of my old friends and started using heroin every day. I am so sick, and I can't stop on my own. I need help."

"We can definitely help you get into rehab. What makes you think you have an infection?"

"A week ago, I started feeling tired and sick. It wasn't a big deal, and I was too busy getting high to notice. That went on for a few days. I started throwing up a couple of days ago. I think I started to run a temperature last night because my teeth kept chattering. Both of my breasts seem swollen and are super tender."

"Would it be alright if I take a look?"

"Sure."

I called in a female nurse into the exam room, and Pam went into the bathroom and undressed. During her undressing, the odor in the room intensified, even from the bathroom. When she came out, she had a gown on. Indeed, both breasts were swollen and red. The redness included the breasts but also the tissue to the side and above. She was very tender and was unable to sit still through my entire exam.

The most surprising aspect of the exam was that she still had a drain from the breast augmentation on both sides of both breasts.

Pam explained, "I haven't seen anyone for follow up after surgery because I was too busy getting high."

"Those drains need to come out."

It took a few minutes to prep the area. I remove the left and right drains, and the result was surprising. Thick, white purulent discharge came spilling out of each wound. The smell was overwhelming. I had to manipulate the skin for several minutes and even cut a wider hole in the skin to get all the discharge expressed.

It was so bad that the patient and the nurse both almost vomited. The infection was much worse than you can imagine. Simple antibiotics were not going to help in the slightest. The infection had gone into the breast tissue and around the implants. Her temperature was 105 degrees, and she was extremely sick.

The nurse quickly began working on setting up an IV site in both arms. We started giving her some pain medications, IV fluids, and something to help with nausea. She wanted to refuse the pain medications because of her addiction history, but she was in such bad shape that she needed them.

A surgical consult was made, and it was determined that each implant needed to be removed. Other providers were consulted, and they came down for their own examinations. She was going to have the tissue debrided of any infection, a wound vac for a few weeks, and possibly reconstructive surgery. It was going to be quite a process.

As they were wheeling her off to be admitted into the hospital, Pam said, "Thank you Dr. Favor for not judging me. I know I made some mistakes, but you looked past my addiction. I appreciate that."

Pam had surgery and remained in the hospital for almost two weeks. She went to rehab and had a few additional surgeries. I happened to see her two years later, and she was doing as good as ever. She had hit rock bottom, twice in fact, and had recognized that she couldn't do this alone. Despite her injuries and addiction, Pam found a way to rebound. The transformation from a homeless and sick patient to a healthy and clean one was remarkable. Sometimes it takes a kind person to help you out of your worst moments.

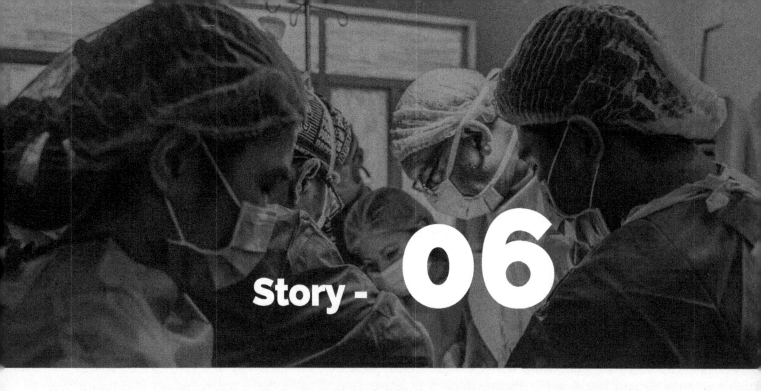

A Potential Disaster in the Emergency Room

In the Emergency Room, you see patients that come and go for whatever specific complaint they may be having. Often, it is a rush of adrenaline for those circumstances where life-saving measures are taken. Sometimes, the adrenaline is the result of the severity or unexpected nature of the injury. Despite these moments, there are plenty of dull times as well. Both aspects of the extremes have both good and bad things that come with them. But day-after-day or hour-after-hour of continuous catastrophic situations often drain even the most prepared of our medical staff.

An area of the ER often overlooked by the casual individual is those select patients who come back repeatedly. In fact, frequently, these individuals may enjoy the ER or the attention they are given. Become a repeat patient could happen because of a variety of reasons, including having a place to stay, getting out of the cold temperatures, social interaction, someone caring for them, severe medical problems, and dozens of other reasons that might make no sense to you or me.

These patients are seen more often than you would expect. For example, the staff might see the same patient five or six times in a month or five or six times a week. These patients often have similar complaints every time they come to the ER, but sometimes they shake it up to see what happens. When it becomes bitter cold or burning hot outside, the ER staff often prepare to see these returning patients. If something serious like an earthquake or other natural disaster occurs, the same thing can be expected.

As frustrating as it might be to have the same patient over and over again, some of them can become part of your ER family - both a good and bad thing. You almost come to expect them and miss them when you haven't seen them for a few months. After six months, you often start worrying about the worst possibilities, and even sometimes, you find that the individual has moved away or died and might never be coming back to the ER. It can be stressful and sad.

This story deals with one such individual. He was a drifter and loved to come to our Emergency Room, especially in the winter. He was homeless and traveled to our warm climate and the beach during the winter to get away from the snow and colder temperatures up north. He was in his sixties and had several health issues. Despite the typically mild weather we had been experiencing, this particular week was different. The weather, even for our city, was downright cold. When the temperature drops this much, even in the desert, everyone starts complaining.

That was when Mr. Davies arrived at the hospital. He came in around five at night, right after the sun had gone down, complaining of a cough, fever, chills, and thought he must have pneumonia. I know he was hoping that we would keep him through dinner and possibly through the night running tests to check for pneumonia and such.

Ninety-Five percent of the time, this man is one of the kindest people you'll ever meet. You must understand that he has some significant mental health issues. The problems start when his paranoia gets really bad. He can be combative when this occurs.

As Mr. Davies was escorted to one of the exam room, I could tell that he wasn't quite himself. He started ranting and raving about how the government was out to get him. The nurse who escorted him was a student, and she had no idea how to control him. The trick is really simple. To help Mr. Davies, you have to also be angry at the government. Tell him that they hassled you, and he will immediately calm. If you argue with him, you might get a punch to the face.

Several of the other nurses recognized his voice, and soon he had three or four people bad mouthing the government. Soon, Mr. Davies was calm and relaxed. The other unbelievable thing about Mr. Davies is that he has a remarkable memory and can remember most of everyone's names. He knows personal information about everyone.

Over the years, we would speculate about why he was homeless in the first place. When he was good, it was really good, but we've also seen the paranoia. The most likely contributing factor to him being homeless is his drinking. The combination of paranoia and drinking likely makes life very difficult for Mr. Davies.

I stopped by his room and heard him asking another nurse about their husband and her three kids. Mr. Davies was wearing three jackets, and it was obvious that they were storing some large bottles of beer. After he was checked in, he admitted he hoped we would give him a room for a few hours and let him drink. We confiscated the alcohol until he was discharged. We weren't really busy and gave him the room for a few hours.

When he awoke, I went into his room, and he was as polite as can be. He answered all the questions. It turned out that he did have a cough and a slight temperature. He said he had felt sick for weeks. Granted - he'd been in the ER twice last week, but nothing was found. This time, he promised me that things had gotten worse. I might have joked about the weather being the only thing that had gotten worse.

By this time, things in the ER had gotten significantly busier. Suddenly, our priorities shifted to a car crash, with multiple people involved. We had some chest pains, broken legs and arms, and numerous other things in the span of the next few hours.

When there was time, the doctor hurried in and saw Mr. Davies and ordered a chest X-ray. The problem was that there were a few people in line for the X-ray machine before Mr. Davies. When I told Mr. Davies that he was going to have to wait, he asked to see the dinner menu. He didn't seem to have a care in the world. I told him that there would be no after-meal drink.

Around midnight, Mr. Davies finally received his X-ray. The chest X-ray showed a small area that might be pneumonia or something else entirely. Mr. Davies was starting to shiver a little from his alcohol withdrawals. We placed an IV and gave him some medications to help. He still wanted to be able to walk around, and I remember him dragging his IV pole down the hall. The doctor decided to get a more specific test on his chest. It would be another hour before it could be done.

After the testing was done, and we were waiting for the results, Mr. Davies informed me that he needed to smoke. I unhooked the IV without removing it, and he grabbed his old jean jacket and went outside. When he finished, he stepped back inside, shivering again. He had smoked one and a half cigarettes. This, he told me, was an improvement. He took the second cigarette and broke off the tip and placed it in his jacket pocket to save it. Back in his room, he removed his coat and lay down on his bed to wait for the results. We got him a bag of crackers and some soda, and he watched some television.

Twenty minutes later, the results still hadn't been processed. I was working in a room next to Mr. Davies when I thought I smelled a faint amount of smoke. My first thought was that a piece of equipment was causing a problem, but then I remember Mr. Davies smoking. It would be my luck to find him smoking in his room. With all the equipment, that would be a disaster.

I sprinted over to his room, picturing the aftermath of an explosion caused by Mr. Davies smoking. Instead, I found him fast asleep. However, the real problem was easy to spot. On the outer edge of the room, Mr. Davies' jacket was on fire. I mean, it was completely ablaze as it hung from a mounted coat rack. The entire bottom half was bright yellow. One of the other staff members grabbed an extinguisher and sprayed out the burning coat before it became the death of us all.

It wasn't hard to assume what had happened. I remembered back to the half cigarette that Mr. Davies had tried to save. I'm convinced that it hadn't been completely extinguished. If Mr. Davies's coat had caught fire in another portion of the hospital, it would've been dire results. Luckily, we have a lot of moving parts, and the coat was quickly discovered.

The best news of the night was that the final diagnosis for Mr. Davies was a normal chest CT. He slept another few hours and was discharged early the next morning. He left with two bottles of beer in his hands and one less jacket.

I've seen Mr. Davies a few times since this all happened, and he loves to tell that story. He embellishes the details to everyone he knows, including all the new staff and anyone who will listen. He laughs and jokes for a dozen minutes or more. Of course, we never allow him to have any cigarettes, a lighter, or alcohol when he comes in through the ER. He can't be trusted.

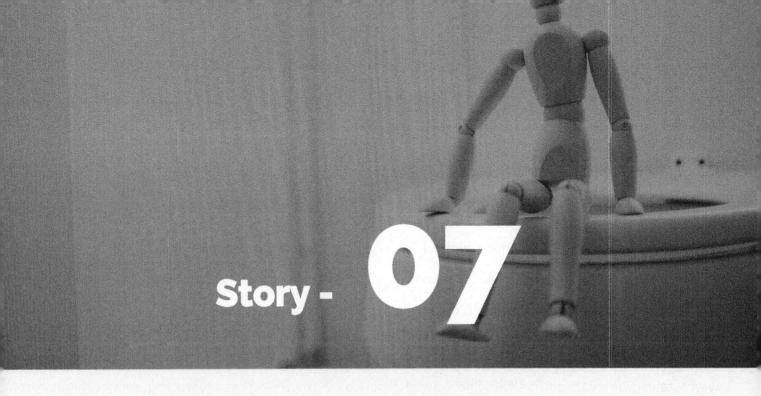

Story - 07

Stuck on the Toilet

A certified nurse assistant (CNA), let's call her Mary, was working in a small community, reporting for her shift at the nursing home. It was the graveyard shift, and she enjoyed this part of the day and this shift. Not everyone can work the graveyard shift, but some do love it. It allowed Mary to study, and she felt she was accomplishing two tasks at once.

She was working in a lockdown unit, which means that anyone coming in or out must be allowed to do so. Typically, they were buzzed in or out. This was especially true for the residents of the nursing home who, unless a prearranged doctor's appointment or family gathering, remained on the unit. At this time of night, no one but the staff was supposed to be going in or out.

Often, there was plenty to do, such as checking on the patients hourly and getting things ready for the next day. Sometimes Mary would need to pass out medications. She was often called to the patient's room for certain questions or to help with bowel movements and more. Additionally, she could do puzzles, play games, watch television, especially before bedtime. Sometimes, a resident wouldn't be able to sleep, and they would come out of their rooms to join Mary or to get some food.

There was a second building for those who did not require a lockdown unit at this particular site. These patients still needed care but to a far less capacity. Another staff person was needed to oversee this second building. They had more patients to monitor, but often, those patients required less work.

After Mary had given the bedtime snack and changed most of the patients, they were sent to their rooms to watch television or to go to sleep. She started cleaning up the dining area, vacuuming and preparing the bedtime medications. She worked for about an hour and had mostly finished everything when the phone rang. On the other end was Fletcher, who was friendly enough but extremely lazy.

Mary answered, "Hello."

"I'm hungry. I am going to go get some pizza. Can you cover my area for like five minutes?" Fletcher asked.

"Now?" she asked. "Didn't you just come on your shift like an hour ago?"

"I'll bring you back half a pizza?"

"I'll be over in five minutes." Reluctantly, Mary agreed; after all, she hadn't brought any food for the night. She finished getting her area ready, locked the doors, and hurried over to the other building. It was nearly eleven at night. When she stepped in, Fletcher was waiting for her.

"There's only one lady to worry about. Her name is Dorothy, and she's in room 112. She's using the restroom. She's here just for a few days. Her family is out of town." He politely added in a softer voice, "She has some problems standing for long periods of time. She is extremely overweight."

Mary nodded and headed down the second hall. She waited for ten minutes for the call light to come on before she stepped inside. When it didn't, she got worried and opened the door. Mary asked, "Dorothy, it's Mary. I am here to help you. Fletcher stepped out for a second. Are you ready?"

Dorothy replied, "Five more minutes."

Five minutes later, the call light came on, and Mary entered the small apartment like bedroom. This unit was especially for more high functioning patients. In Dorothy's case, like many others, she was there for a short time only. Her family was the primary caregiver. Since they had gone out of town, Dorothy needed a place to stay. As far as Mary knew, this was the first time Dorothy had come to visit. Many other patients had come over the years; some had been following a stroke and release from a hospital. Others had a hip fracture and needed a few weeks of recovery. Dorothy was like many other patients before her.

As Mary entered, Dorothy said, "I am in the bathroom. Can you help me stand up?"

Mary continued to the bathroom and found Dorothy finished with the toilet. Fletcher had been right, Dorothy was overweight. She was likely over 400 pounds. Again, it was not unusual for this type of patient to come to the nursing home.

Dorothy said, "So sorry to ask for your help, dear."

Mary stepped into the doorway. "Don't worry. This is what we do, and I love my job."

"Well, I absolutely hate this part. It's so embarrassing."

The bathroom was small. The doorway was to the right of the room. The toilet was followed by the sink, and in the back corner was a small standup shower without a bathtub. Mary stepped inside and tried using her hands, interlaced with Dorothy's hands, to get her up from the toilet. That didn't work.

Dorothy added, "I guess I'm really stuck."

"No worries," Mary said. "Let me come to your side, and I'll trying to reach under your shoulder and help you up."

Unfortunately, that didn't work either. The last option was to give Dorothy a bear hug, wrapping her arms around her. Dorothy agreed. Mary reached under both arms and reached around Dorothy. It took a few attempts, but with Dorothy trying to stand and Mary pulling her up, she finally stood.

That was when the real problems started. Dorothy had been sitting too long, and her legs had gone numb. With Mary still guiding her, Dorothy tried taking a few small steps, but her pants and underwear were still down at her ankles. Dorothy tripped forward and crashed into Mary. Luckily, Mary was able to maneuver correctly, and they didn't smash into the wall. Instead, Dorothy fell forward as Mary fell backward. They fell through the open doorway, and Dorothy ended up landing on top of Mary, who provided the cushion in the fall.

"Are you hurt?" Mary asked after the dust had settled. (Actually, it was a whole lot of baby powder)

Dorothy refused to answer.

Mary took the next few minutes to assess the situation. She was completely stuck, unable to move at all.

"Roll to the side, and I might be able to get out," Mary encouraged.

Still, Dorothy was unable to respond.

Mary took a moment to catalog her own injuries. The back of her head had hit the floor, and she had started to bleed. Her left arm was still caught awkwardly underneath Dorothy. She remembered Fletcher but realized he had only left a few minutes ago. He was likely going to be gone another several minutes. She couldn't reach the call line, and even if she could, what would that accomplish? She decided to give Dorothy a few minutes to recover.

Five minutes later, Dorothy began to sob. Mary felt so bad for her, but her own arm was starting to cramp. Mary began to yell, but at the same time, trying to be encouraging, "Dorothy. I know we can do this. I know we can get out of this. If we work together, we can get out of this."

For the first time, Dorothy spoke, through her sobs, "What do you want me to do?"

"You'll have to roll to your left, so I can get my arm out."

"I think I can do that."

Dorothy rolled, and it took a few long minutes, but Mary was able to finally release her arm. It felt so good to be able to move her arm again. Mary said, "Great job. Now let's have you roll to your right; I think that will free me enough." It took another five minutes before Mary was able to pull herself out.

Halfway through, Dorothy started to cry again. She said, "This is the most embarrassing thing that's ever happened to me."

"And it's over. Never to worry about it again," Mary said as she stood.

It took a while to get Dorothy dressed, into a wheelchair and moved over to her bed. It wasn't hard to get her back into bed and settled. Mary sat with Dorothy for several minutes and talked. Mary learned a lot about Dorothy's personal life, favorite foods, and movies. It wasn't long before they were good friends.

Fletcher came back after another twenty minutes. In all, he was gone for almost an hour. But Mary never said anything to Fletcher about Dorothy or what had really happened. The worst part, he didn't even bring back any pizza with him.

Mary continued to visit Dorothy every day for the next two weeks before Dorothy left. It turned out to be a difficult but good experience for both of them.

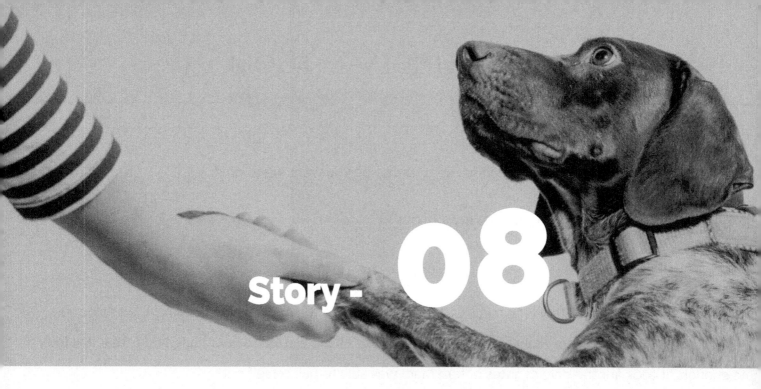

Patient in Jail Acting Very Unusual - He was Missing his Dog

Treating unusual individuals in jail is not unexpected. Sometimes it has something to do with their mental health, medical health, or something entirely different. Sometimes you see things because of drug use, withdrawals, anger, manipulation, and much more. In some cases, when they act "normally," that's when we become concerned. We have over 1500 inmates in our jail at any given time. Treating all of them, at times, can be challenging for our medical staff.

One individual who had been in jail for a few days started acting quite a bit different than when he arrived. Day one, he had an intake screening and spoke with the nurse for an hour or more. He had just a few medications, and those were sent to our intake director, a physician, for approval. They were approved and ordered. He showered and changed into his new jail clothing. A detailed medical assessment was done, including his medical history, risk factors, previous injuries, mental health history, and previous drug use.

I think he thought he was going to bail out and believed he wasn't going to be in jail for only a few hours.

On his nursing intake assessment, he reported he had no medical issues or other concerns. He had his wisdom teeth out when he was back in high school. He had no other surgeries or such. He had no history of drug use and told the staff that there was minimal risk of any medical problems or withdrawal. He was placed in housing and was monitored.

That night, he began calling the nurses and asking to see the officers every hour. At one point during the night, he became anxious about his dog. He described the dog to every staff member he came across. To the nurses, he asked to be released from jail to be able to go take care of his dog. He also wanted repeat phone calls so that his family would go check on his house. He ended up getting very little sleep that first night.

From that point, he started to get more and more anxious. He wasn't sleeping and started freaking out every hour or so. The staff tried helping him in any way they could. He was given showers, medications, and several other things to help, including books, paper, pencils, and more.

Soon mental health was called to his cell because of his behavior. In one moment, he would refuse to eat or see anyone, and in the next instant, he was demanding to see the president. No one could understand what was happening. His issues and complaints were jumping from one thing to another. He began crying about his family, his job, his dog, a high-school girlfriend that he hadn't seen in ten years, and even the Cleveland Browns' football team.

Finally, he was placed on the provider's clinic and was called down to the exam room for a medical visit.

The patient, Jacob, was so distressed that he was brought to his appointment in a wheelchair. With the help of two officers, we placed him on the exam table. He talked to an imaginary person sitting inside the wall and had trouble responding to my questions. His vitals and behavior were reviewed. Nothing about his current behavior made any sense. I was able to do a full exam, and besides his behavior, everything was normal. I called a few pharmacies, but he didn't have any known mental health medications. In the end, I could only come up with one thing –drug withdrawal.

I asked, "Hey, Jacob. Have you ever used Meth, Heroin, or another drug?"

Jacob answered quickly, "No, doc. I don't use that crap stuff."

"Do you smoke marijuana, spice, vape, or any mixture of things?"

"I can promise you that I've never smoked a joint or shot anything up. Vaping is for losers, and I am not a loser."

"I believe you. I'm just trying to understand why your behavior has changed so much over the last few days."

"I don't want to be in jail."

I laughed. "Most people don't. Where do you want to be?"

"At home with my family. Did I tell you that my family is sick?"

"I don't think you did."

"Really sick. Like in a bad way."

"Who's sick? What's going on?"

"My dog is so sick. Her name is Lucy, and she has cancer."

"That's horrible. What kind of dog? How old is she?"

"She is like eight. She is a basset hound. I think she has something like lymphoma."

(At this point, I was pretty amazed at how well he was talking. He had a great recall of events, dogs, names, and remembering lymphoma was pretty astonishing. Most patients can't remember what medications they take.)

I said, "That's terrible. How is she doing?"

"She's dying. The chemo isn't working."

"I'm sorry. That would make me want to get out of jail too. I bet you're stressed."

"Exactly. No one will listen to me. Can't you just let me go?"

"No. Sorry. The medical staff can't let you out of jail."

"Who's going to give my dog her meds?"

"Have you called a family member?"

"Sure. But they don't want to light up the pot grass I have at home."

This peeked my attention. "What is the pot grass?"

"Something, my friend gave me. He told me that it would work well to help my dog feel more comfortable and take away her pain."

"What is it that you do with it?"

"I close all the windows, and I light up this pouch of the stuff. The room gets kind of smoky. It is so relaxing and makes me and my dog pretty hungry. I also spray this oil under her tongue several times a day. I've tried it a few times as well."

"Like CBD oil or something."

"Maybe," Jacob said.

"How often do you light up the pot grass?"

"Few times a day. It really helps me to calm myself down."

"Good to know."

"Do you use any other herbal products?"

"I don't think so, doc."

"I think we can help you."

"Get out?"

"No. Just to feel better."

"Hey look. There's my uncle Fester. Didn't he die like five years ago?"

I turned around, but there was no one else in the room with us. The officers began laughing uncontrollably.

At some point, I ended the visit, and Jacob was moved to withdrawal monitoring. Heavy use of marijuana and CBD oil can cause this type of side effects in some patients. Sometimes it can get so bad that you can start hallucinating. Jacob was given some IV fluids and some medications and recovered just fine. Our medical staff checked on him every day. About four days later, he had completely forgotten our previous conversation. He was far more rational and calmer.

There were no mental health problems, just using some marijuana and CBD oil from his friend to help his dog. That part turned out to be entirely true. I tried explaining that he needed to look for a better treatment for his dog, but I was pretty confident that he would shut the blinds and light up a pouch the moment he was released from jail.

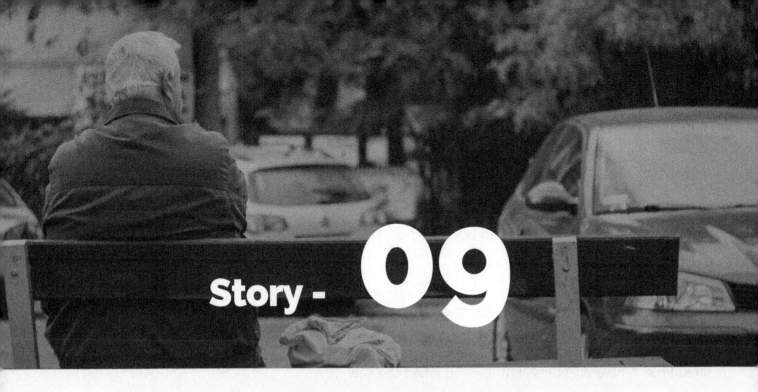

Story - 09

Escaped Resident from a Nursing Home

After dinner, I often sit down with some of the nursing home residents to play games or listen to stories. One night, after serving dinner, I sat down with George to hear about another, more private story he wanted to share. He was starting to have symptoms of Dementia, and he would forget things, get angry, and have trouble problem-solving. But, when his memory was in top shape, he would tell some of the most amazing stories. And today was a good day for Mr. Myers.

George Myers was a great storyteller. Even at dinner, he had told some of the ladies some of the amazing things he had done when he was younger. He used hand gestures, winks, smiles, and plenty of passion. He had the entire room captivated. It was a good day, and the entire room was laughing.

His mind was as clear as I had seen it in months. Another resident had recently died, and the mood had been somber for weeks. But today, it felt like maybe things were changing for the better.

An hour later, I was called to a resident's room to help with a shower. This is a typical function of our staff, and several patients get their showers at night. As I finished getting the resident dressed, an alarm went off, signaling that one of the doors had been opened. This was only to happen in emergencies. I quickly finished what I was doing and ran to the lobby.

Amber, the LPN in charge for the night, was frantic. She was sending two other nursing assistants around to each room to make sure that everyone was reassured and calmed. Rich and I arrived in the lobby around the same time. Amber was tense but relieved when she saw us.

Pointing to the side door, Amber said, "Mr. Myers just got into a fight with another resident and took off running. You guys need to go find him and bring him back."

I said, "Call the police if we're not back in ten minutes."

Rich and I headed out the door. We're located in a somewhat busy area of town. Right outside the door is an open parking lot. Behind us is a fair number of trees. I didn't think that he would wander through the forest.

Rich said, "I'll head up the street, and you go down."

I said, "Sounds good to me."

"Call if you see anything."

We headed off in different directions. I sprinted through the parking lot, and when I reached the street, I turned right. I ran down a block and found Mr. Myers' shoe in the middle of the sidewalk. I called back to Rich and Amber and told them what I found. Rich was going to double back - on a different street, just in case. I continued forward.

Another block down, I ran into a girl who was really upset. She was on the phone, and I heard a bit of her conversation. She was upset about this man who had just run by. I hurried over to her and tapped her on the shoulder. When she turned, I asked, "Did you just say something about an old man?"

She held up a shirt, and I recognized it as Mr. Myers'. She added, "Yea, you did. It was crazy. He ran up to me, took off his shirt, and started dancing for me. He tried to kiss me. I pushed him away, and he laughed and threw his shirt at me."

"Which way did he go?" I asked, taking the shirt.

She pointed further down the street, and I sprinted off. I found his sock near a restaurant. Glancing in the window, it wasn't surprising to find that half of the guests were on their feet, quite angry. As I stepped inside, it didn't take long to learn that a half-naked man ran through the restaurant knocking down several drinking glasses. I scrambled to the back door that led into the alley, but it was empty. There was a commotion ahead, and I continued running forward.

This time, I found another woman ranting. I paused to asked, "Was it a half-naked older man?"

"He kissed me. Like three times."

"Sorry about that. He has some medical issues. Do you know where he went?"

She pointed down a different street that went almost perpendicular to the one he was on. I called Rich and Amber and told them what was happening. Amber said that she was going to call the manager so that the restaurant could be called, and the situation was explained. I took off running.

A block later, I found some underwear on the ground. That was not a good sign.

Screams down another side street told me exactly where to find Mr. Myers. I called Rich, and he was going to return to the nursing home and get the van. I ran the last few hundred feet, unsure of what I was going to find. What I witnessed was a total shock, Mr. Myers was near a well-known hotel. He was still wearing a single sock and a shoe on one foot. He was completely naked otherwise. He was lying on a car, on a taxi, on the front window, spread eagle. Luckily, there were no passengers inside. The driver, however, was standing outside of the car and yelling at Mr. Myers. Several of the hotel's patrons were laughing, screaming, and pointing.

When I reached the car, the driver was trying to pull Mr. Myers off the car. I hurried forward and explained what was going on. It took a full minute to get Mr. Myers' attention. By now, he was tired, and all the energy was out of him. He let me help him off the car. I don't think he recognized me in the slightest. He allowed me to guide him to the grass. He sat down, and I started to put on his shirt and his underwear. I even put on the second shoe. His pants, I have no idea what he did with them.

Rich arrived with the van a few minutes later. We got Mr. Myers inside and back to the nursing home. A few weeks later, he was transferred to a lockdown facility. This had been his third time running from our facility, and we could no longer handle him. But Mr. Myers and his stories of adventure would surely be missed. In the end, restitution was made at the restaurant, and everyone had a good story to tell.

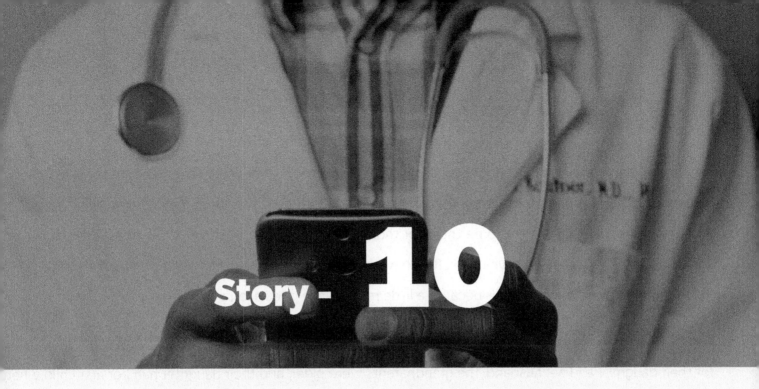

Story - **10**

A Phone Call to the Pediatrician about an Oven

Life in a pediatric clinic can be exciting and rewarding. Watching and treating children from the beginning is such an unbelievable experience. It is like having the excitement of the parent without the same responsibility. To watch a child's growth, achievements, and successes and see the happiness on the faces of their parents, siblings, caregivers, or whoever brings them in, is indescribable.

But, on the same token, when something goes horribly wrong such as cancer, hormone problems, injuries, and such, the heart-tugging seems to be so much stronger. I love working with children but could never treat only sick patients with such things as cancer or incurable disease. I need to see the happiness, growth, and accomplishments of these children.

We all know that potential injuries and problems for children can occur at any time of the day. In fact, some of the craziest injuries happen we've seen happen in the afternoons, evenings, and on weekends. For that reason, we have many of our staff on call - to receive these types of phone calls. Truth be told, some families use this on-call program for just about everything. They called for tooth pains when teething, or a slight rash, or when cramping during their daughter's first menstrual period. Each of us handles medicine and pain differently, and our clinic wants to be there for those types of questions. Some of the questions are absurd and unreasonable. Other calls have been after they waited longer than they should have. We want to be there for all of these types of phone calls because a little reassurance goes a long way.

On a weekend in February, I received a series of phone calls from a set of grandparents who were babysitting for their daughter and her husband. The grandparents were older, and their daughter had her first child when she was older as well. This meant that it had been years since the grandparents had young children in the home, and they had forgotten quite a bit. They didn't want to bother their daughter while she was on vacation in Hawaii. She had just received a job advancement and pay raise, and a vacation was sorely needed.

The grandparents were watching their ten-month-old granddaughter. The first phone call came from the grandfather. It was about a rash that had started on the abdomen of the baby. It was red and splotchy. This is a common appearance of a rash for a child of this age. It could be something they ate, like an allergy - especially if new foods are being introduced. It could be a virus if the child is in daycare. It also could be a variety of other things such as heat rash, diaper rash, or something else entirely.

I spent half an hour on the phone, answering several different questions. I should've spotted some of the problems at this point. It was apparent that the grandparents were clueless about too many things. They were starting to freak out. I reassured them and told them to send me a picture of the rash. When it came, the rash was very minimal. I texted back and recommended a bath, some lotion, and a change of clothes a few times a day. They were relieved and grateful for the reassurance I gave.

The next day, the grandmother called. She was really scared. I could hear it in her voice. The rash had progressed and was now on the cheeks of the baby girl. She was fussy, and the rash was much more pronounced than the day before. She reported that there was a small amount of redness on the arms and on the chest that still remained. Again, pictures were sent. Also, the grandmother confirmed that daycare was being used by her daughter.

From the photos and history, it appeared to be Fifths Disease - a contagious rash that is caused by a virus - Parvovirus B19. I reassured the grandmother at length. She didn't seem quite convinced but listened. I suggested some Tylenol as needed. The grandmother assured me that they had some liquid Tylenol, and I instructed on how to give the right amount.

As I hung up the phone, I said, "Remember to take her temperature and tell me if it gets over 100.4 degrees."

The grandmother replied, "No problem. Will do."

The next phone call, the third, came later that night. This time, it was the grandfather who was speaking. It was as if he was on speakerphone. He asked, "How do we take our granddaughter's temperature. My wife says she feels really hot."

"Do you have a thermometer?"

"I am not sure what it looks like."

I said, "They are usually white. One end is fatter. The other end is skinnier and goes in the child's mouth or under their arm or in their bum."

"Did you say in their bum?"

"Yep. There are thermometers that do that."

"I don't see any of those. But I don't really know what I am looking for."

(You must understand that at this time, a few years ago, we didn't have the internet to check on the pictures of medical things. We also didn't have the thermometers that you can run across the forehead. We did have the ones, in our clinic, that you put in the ears. Most families at home had the simple mercury thermometers or some that read the temperature.)

From the background, I heard, "Told you. We don't have a choice."

The voice of the grandfather changed; it became more frantic. He asked, "Is there another way to check a temperature?"

"You can feel their forehead with your hand to see if it is warmer. It won't give you an accurate reading, but you can try."

The grandfather screamed, "STOP!"

I wasn't sure if he was talking to me. I asked, "Did I say something?"

Again, the voice of the grandmother could be heard, "Why are you yelling at me? We need to check the temperature; this is the only way."

"Not a good idea," said the grandfather.

At this point, I was really confused.

The grandfather said, back into the phone, "Tell me your experience of using the oven to check the temperature. My wife has turned it on to 100 degrees. She thinks that the baby will cry if she doesn't have a temperature, and we put her inside for a few minutes."

I screamed, "Absolutely not. That's a terrible idea. Do not put her in the oven."

The grandmother asked, "Are you sure? It seems logical."

"It's not. In fact, why don't you bring the child to my office right now? I will check her out, and we can take her temperature together."

The grandfather said, "You would really be willing to do that at this time of night?"

"Oh yes," I reassured them. "It wouldn't be a problem at all. In fact, I was already heading in to do some paperwork."

It turned out to be fifth's disease, the virus. It cleared up after another several days. I spent an hour quizzing the grandparents about what to do if such and such happened. They answered all the questions correctly. I gave them a thermometer and showed them how it worked. They called again after their babysitting journey was over and promised that they had learned their lesson. I mean, who thinks sticking a child in the oven is the right thing to do?

Made in the USA
Las Vegas, NV
01 July 2021